Reversing Ectropion: I

C000319329

The Raw Vegan Plant-Based Di Regeneration Workbook for Healing Patients.

Volume 4

Health Central

Copyright © 2019

Deficiencies & Absorption

"DEFICIENCIES are to blame" says Mr Porter (Dietician) to his patient, Albert.

For argument's sake let's assume that the dietician is correct, and that deficiencies are to blame for Albert's sickness.

Could it then be due to Albert's food being deficient in nutrition? He eats a variety of foods daily, including fresh fruits and vegetables, but yet he is still "deficient" in all the main vitamins and minerals. How could this be?

Many professionals from within the health sector offer questionable dietary ("eat more meat for protein") and supplement ("take Chromium for your Pancreas") advice to patients. Sadly this advice is based on a misguided premise – with treatment, and not cure, being the goal.

If you are advised that your conditions are due to deficiencies then you are not being presented with the complete picture - because if indeed you are deficient, there is a deeper issue at play.

If you are eating foods that are loaded with vitamins and minerals but yet you are still low on them – it is easy to be misled into thinking that your diet is unhealthy.

However we should first look at the root causes and their related factors. The foundation stone of your body is its terrain. So for example if the processes of digestion, absorption, utilisation, and healthy elimination of your waste are hindered, this will eventually create problems for you.

In order to correct absorption issues, we must first understand how the lymphatic system works. Additionally, an understanding of utilisation is necessary. Without these tools, you will risk remaining constipated (both mentally and physically) whilst ignoring the causative factors of your health challenges.

Now that we understand that everything stems from the terrain of your body, our focus is turned towards removing the congested sewage that blocks the flow of energy in relation to eliminating effectively.

The removal of damaging acid from the body is vital for your key glands to recover and resume utilisation of consumed nutrition, vitamins and minerals.

All too often we find the small intestines of our patients to be interstitially (deep within cells and tissues) damaged with acids, and their large intestines (and colon) are plastered with mucoid plaque. This is the root cause of poor absorption of nutrition and this means that you will not receive the full benefits from your consumed foods. This also means that taking supplements will not yield the results that you desire. Instead, they will only worsen the issue and over-stimulate and acidify your body.

You Must...

Your lymphatic system needs to be flushed out in order for your absorption and utilisation to start working for you again. This sewage system is your body's main elimination backbone, and is responsible for cleansing your blood and organs of accumulated acids and waste.

Acids damage the soft tissue infrastructure within your body. If the foods that you consume are acidic, regardless of them being full of "nutrition", you will continue to suffer from cell damage and a breakdown of your eliminative organs (kidneys, bowels, skin, lungs). This will lead to waste backing up within your different systems, which will cause damage to organs such as the adrenal glands which are responsible for mineral utilisation.

Your adrenal glands also work hand-in-hand with the kidneys, and with the adrenal glands struggling, your kidneys will lose their ability to effectively filter and remove the acids out of your lymphatic system.

As you can see, your body is built up of an interconnected system which needs to be corrected systemically.

We want to target the root causes by cleansing the body's sewage clearing system, correct digestion, absorption, utilization and eliminate accumulated metabolitic waste, along with any hidden old faecal matter waste from previous poor dietary habits.

We also need to remove mucus through our eliminative organs whilst also removing the destructive acids that are responsible for breaking down tissues, which effectively leads to internal dysfunction and eventual dis-ease.

How?

We must start by becoming conscious and aware of the destructive foods that we are actively eating on a daily basis. All cooked foods with their energy sapping nature, along with the added chemicals which cause damage to your organs, and central and autonomic nervous systems - must be removed from your routine.

You will also need to remove the following from your day-to-day lifestyle in order to make positive healing gains:

a) Genetically Modified Organisms (GMOs) – e.g. corn, soy.

b) all neuro-toxic pesticide-immersed foods,

c) all chemical-based skin products, and breathable toxic chemicals,

d) fluoride water used for drinking and bathing in (use a filter instead),

e) eliminate the combined consumption of wheat and animal products - it is these that contribute mostly towards disturbing your absorption and utilisation.

A variety of acidic and sub-acidic fruits, including berries, melons, citrus, will all promote the cleansing of your lymphatic system, and support you in opening up your eliminative organs and related endocrine glands.

We MUST make a gradual transition from your current diet (by eliminating the dehydrating foods) and start introducing a raw fruit-based diet which is hydrating, cleansing and full of biologically available nutrition for your cells. With any transition, the secret is to support your adrenal glands, kidneys, and digestive organs.

When you finally start absorbing effectively, you will find that you actually do not require large portions in order to feel strong and full of energy.

If you are at the extreme end of sickness - I would recommend moving into a pure juiced fruit regimen, incorporating herbal and glandular formulas to help you transition from a previous diet (it can be quite a shock and stressful for the body when moving over to a fully raw diet). Vegetable juices will also support your organs through this phase.

Helpful Notes

The subject of transitioning over from a standard diet to a raw fruit diet is a delicate one and if not done correctly, you will experience some challenges.

However, this is normal because considering that your body is congested from your regular dietary routine – to now having a detoxifying diet will mean that your body will send out a variety of signals due to it no longer being fed what it had become accustomed to.

During this phase of transition, based on experience with our patients, we recommend that you support the following organs:

1. The Pituitary Gland (PG) stimulates its fellow endocrine glands (Thyroid, Parathyroid, Adrenal, Pancreas, Gonads, Pineal). So if the PG is down – the other related glands will also likely be suffering. In order to support the PG, we typically use pituitary glandular formulas for chronic patients, and herbs (tincture form being preferred initially) that promote healthy brain and nerve blood circulation (e.g. Gingko, Hawthorn Berry). For dosage information, you must start off small and work up to what feels comfortable for you.

2. The Parathyroid Gland regulates calcium utilisation and for effective calcium uptake into the body, and strong bones, we need to ensure that the calcium that we are consuming from food is being put to work otherwise there will be an imbalance and the stagnant acids in your lymphatic system will pinch the calcium from your bones, resulting in weaker bones (and varicose veins, brain herniation, anxiety, depression, spider veins, brittle fingernails, low calcium levels, bone spurs, fibroids, hemorrhoids, osteoporosis, scoliosis, arthritis, prolapsing of organs).

For optimal parathyroid function, we must ensure that the lymphatic system is being flushed out of acids through a high fruit regimen, whilst maintaining a decent level of calcium through the diet. The herbs Horsetail and Alfalfa are rich in calcium. Sea moss is also very good.

3. The Adrenal Glands (sat right on top of your kidneys) are responsible for sugar metabolisation and mineral utilisation. These glands are yet another set of organs that we find patients to be struggling with.

When moving over to a high fruit diet, the adrenal glands can struggle to cope with the high levels of sugar. You will also find that the change in diet will cause a slight stress response from your adrenal glands, which can then lead to many symptoms – a common one being an increased salt craving.

However, you must continue to push forward as this will be short-lived because a high fruit diet will flush out your whole urinary tract, including your adrenal glands and kidneys.

Some of the herbs that will help in supporting your adrenal glands are Parsley, Kelp, Licorice Root, Cleavers, Saw Palmetto, Dandelion Root.

4. Your Kidneys (including your skin – the 3rd kidney) are the most important eliminative organs within your lymphatic system. The acidic lymph waste will leave your body through these avenues, so it is crucial that we are taking care of them.

Again, a hydrating and cleansing high fruit diet will help to wash out your kidneys, and the addition of herbs will support your progress. Some of the herbs that we use for improving kidney health include: Uva Ursi, Parsley, and Stinging Nettle Leaf.

5. Intestines/Colon – many recommend enemas and colonics and although we are not opposed to these practices every so often, we prefer to focus on our methodology of improving health from the cellular level. Besides fruits such as grapes, mangos, prunes, figs – the herbs that we use to support a deep gut cleanse include Cascara Sagrada (gentle laxative) and Slippery Elm Bark (lubricates the gut).

Physical things to do that we have found to work

1. Sweating with a sauna or in a hot climate helps with the elimination of acids.

2. Raising vitamin D levels naturally through exposure to sunlight also contributes towards healing.

3. Deep breathing exercises by the sea (or any other "off-grid" fresh environment) are vital for the acceleration of your healing. Oxygen has a huge part to play in good health and the deterrence of dis-ease.

4. If you are able to do so, jumping on the rebounder/trampoline is a highly recommended way of moving your lymphatic fluid. Start off jumping for as long as is comfortable and work up to 15 to 20 minutes per day. As you progress, you can try out different jumping techniques.

Finally...

Our goal is to remove acids from your body whilst hydrating and alkalizing it. A fruit diet, with some vegetables from time to time, combined with intermittent dry fasting is the way to achieve this.

Let's tackle the root causes and empower our health to a frequency of high vibration and electricity so our bodies normalise and become dis-ease free.

Good luck – stay focused – remain persistent - it really is easy.

Wishing you all the best and if you would like to book a consultation or have any queries, thoughts, feedback / comments, feel free to email us at:

HealingCentral8@gmail.com

Good Luck with your healing journey.

The Power of Journaling

Journaling your inner self talk is a truly effective way of increasing self awareness and consciousness. To be able to transfer your thoughts and feelings onto a piece of paper is a really effective method of self reflection and improvement. This is much needed when you are switching to a high fruit dietary routine.

You are welcome to add notes on any spaces you find within this book – or alternatively you can use a basic notepad. Be sure to add the date of journaling at the top of each page used. This is invaluable for when you wish to go back and review your feelings and thoughts on previous dates.

Keep a comprehensive record of activities, thoughts, and really log everything you ate/are eating. You can even make miscellaneous notes if you feel that they will help you.

I like to use journals to have a conversation with myself. Inner talk can really help you overcome any challenges that you are experiencing. Express yourself and any concerns that you may have.

Try to advise yourself as though you are your best friend – similarly to how you would advise a close friend or family member. You will be surprised at the results that you will achieve from using this technique.

We have laid out the following examples of different ways that you could complete your daily journaling with the support of this book. These are just basic examples – you can complete your daily journals in any other way that you feel is most comfortable for you.

Tried & Tested Fruit Juicer: **YourFruitJuicer.com**
Tried & Tested Vegetable Juicer: **YourVegJuicer.com**

Got Meaty/Starchy/Cheesey Food Cravings?
CureMyParasite.com

[EXAMPLE 1]
Today's Date: 6th May 2018

Morning

I just ate 3 mangoes - very sweet and tasty. I felt a heavy feeling under my chest area so I stopped eating. Unsure what that was - maybe digestive or the transverse colon?

Afternoon

I was feeling hungry so I am eating some dried figs, pineapple and apricots with around 750ml of spring water.

Evening

Sipping on a green tea (herbal). Feeling pretty strong and alert at the moment.

Night

Enjoying a bowl of red seeded grapes. Currently I feel satisfied.

Today's Notes (Highlights, Thoughts, Feelings):

Unlike yesterday, today was a good day. I am noticing an increase in regular bowel movements which makes me feel cleansed and light afterwards. I feel as though my kidneys are also starting to filter better (white sediment visible in morning wee).

It definitely helps to document my thoughts in this workbook. A great way to reflect, improve and stay on track.

Feeling very good - vibrant and strong - I have noticed a major improvement in my physical fitness and performance. Mentally I feel healthier and happier.

[EXAMPLE 2]
Today's Date: 7th May 2018

Morning

Dry fasting (water and food free since 8pm last night) - will go up until 12:30pm today, and start with 500ml of spring water before eating half a watermelon.

Afternoon

Kept busy and was in and out quite a bit – so nothing consumed.

Evening

At around 5pm, I had a peppermint tea with a selection of mixed dried fruit (small bowl of apricot, dates, mango, pineapple, and prunes).

Night

Sipped on spring water through the evening as required.
Finished off the other half of the watermelon from the morning.

Today's Notes (Highlights, Thoughts, Feelings):

As with most days, today started well with me dry fasting (continuing my fast from my sleep/skipping breakfast) up until around 12:30pm and then eating half a watermelon. The laxative effect of the watermelon helped me poop and release any loosened toxins from the fasting period.
I tend to struggle on some days from 3pm onwards. Up until that point I am okay but if the cravings strike then it can be challenging. I remind myself that those burgers and chips do not have any live healing energy.
I feel good in general. I feel fantastic doing a fruit/juice fast but slightly empty by the end of the day.
Cooked food makes me feel severe fatigue and mental fog.
Will continue with my fruit fasting and start to introduce fruit juices due to their deeper detox benefits. I would love to be on juices only as I have seen others within the community achieve amazing results.

[EXAMPLE 3]
Today's Date: 8th May 2018

Morning

Today I woke and my children were enjoying some watermelon for breakfast – and the smell was luring so I joined them. Large bowl of watermelon eaten at around 8am. Started with a glass of water.

Afternoon

Snacked on left over watermelon throughout the morning and afternoon. Had 5 dates an hour or so after.

Evening

Had around 3 mangoes at around 6pm. Felt content – but then I was invited round to a family gathering where a selection of pizzas, burgers and chips were being served. I gave into the peer pressure and felt like I let myself down!

Night

Having over-eaten earlier on in the evening, I was still feeling bloated with a headache (possibly digestion related) and I also felt quite mucus filled (wheez in chest and coughing up phlegm). Very sleepy and low energy. The perils of cooked foods!!

Today's Notes (Highlights, Thoughts, Feelings):

I let myself down today. It all started well until I ate a fully blown meal (and over-ate). I didn't remain focussed and I spun off track. As a result my energy levels were much lower and I felt a bout of extreme fatigue 30 minutes after the meal (most likely the body struggling to with digesting all that cooked food).
I need to stick to the plan because the difference between fruit fasting, and eating cooked foods is huge – 1 makes you feel empowered whilst the other makes you feel drained. I also felt the mucus overload after the meal – it kicked in pretty quickly.
Today I felt disappointed after giving in to the meal but tomorrow is a new day and I will keep on going! It is important to remind myself that I won't get better if I cannot stick to the routine.

Frequently Asked Questions

1. Does dry fasting involve not showering or brushing my teeth?
Not entirely but some do take it to this level. We simply recommend
that you work up towards not eating or drinking for prolonged periods
(18+ hours) - ideally from the previous night until the evening before
breaking your fast with dates, prune juice, grapes, oranges - or any
other laxative based fruit that you enjoy.

2. What if my sodium and potassium levels drop down on a fruit diet?
Initially, going from a standard diet, your organs will not be completely
prepared to respond to the full force of fruits. This is where you will
need to strengthen any weak organs such as the adrenal glands,
kidneys, and various digestive organs - so that absorption and
utilisation can take place efficiently and your body is supported
through this dietary transition. An Iris Diagnosis can also highlight
your main weaknesses.

**3. My friend recommended that I take part in Ramadan and fast for a
whole month with her. She said I will feel more present-minded and
I will have a feeling of accountability. Is this a good idea?**
Yes. Any type of prolonged dry fasting will yield beneficial results
however do note that you must break the fast with a laxative based fruit
(dates, prunes, figs), followed by fruits that are kind to your kidneys
(oranges, grapes, melons) and will support them through filtration.
With fasting, we must focus on the elimination organs because fasting
itself starves off weak/damaged cells and accumulates toxins, ready for
disposal. These need to be disposed of gently during the fast opening
period. Additionally, any type accountability is a good idea because it
will keep you on track to reach your goals. **Note:** if you are fasting for
the first time, ensure you are supporting your kidneys with herbs and/
or glandulars.

4. Is it true that disease starts at the colon?
I would say that to reverse a chronic condition, you must start by
cleansing your lower digestive system which includes the intestines
and colon. The kidneys also play a vital role in this process. We have
found that the most chronic patients have one thing in common - they
all have a deeply congested colon. I would recommend using an enema
irregularly, drink the cold-pressed juice of plums (or dates, grapes,
prunes, figs) and take herbs such as Cascara Sagrada, and Slippery Elm
Bark.
For fruit juicing: **YourFruitJuicer.com**
For vegetable juicing: **YourVegJuicer.com**

DAY STRUCTURE REMINDERS

For The Morning...

Continuing your dry fast from your night sleep is a good idea. Work towards fasting up until at least 12pm. As your body adapts, start to increase this - the later you break your fast - the better.

In The Afternoon...

When you do finally decide to open your fast - focus on hydration. Spring water is a good start or slow-juiced fruits (e.g. berries, melons, citrus). Alternatively, eating soaked dates or your favourite fruits will suffice.

Evening Feast...

Work towards dry fasting for 23 hours and eating for 1 hour each day. This will take time to reach - listen to your body and get there in your own pace. The ideal time to break your dry fast would be approximately 6pm to 7pm

And At Night Time...

Be sure to completely stop eating by 8pm (latest) so your body can prepare for a good night's sleep, rest and recovery.

DAY 1: DAILY TIP

"Get yourself an accountability partner to complete a 30 day detox with.

Start with 7 days and work your way up.

It will be fun and motivating completing it with somebody (or a group) ...or of course you can go it alone."

DAY STRUCTURE REMINDERS

For The Morning...
Continuing your dry fast from your night sleep is a good idea. Work towards fasting up until at least 12pm. As your body adapts, start to increase this - the later you break your fast - the better.

In The Afternoon...
When you do finally decide to open your fast - focus on hydration. Spring water is a good start or slow-juiced fruits (e.g. berries, melons, citrus). Alternatively, eating soaked dates or your favourite fruits will suffice.

Evening Feast...
Work towards dry fasting for 23 hours and eating for 1 hour each day. This will take time to reach - listen to your body and get there in your own pace. The ideal time to break your dry fast would be approximately 6pm to 7pm

And At Night Time...
Be sure to completely stop eating by 8pm (latest) so your body can prepare for a good night's sleep, rest and recovery.

"Remember when starting out, it is important to keep yourself hydrated throughout the day. Spring Water is a good start - and slow/cold pressed juice is also very powerful."

DAY STRUCTURE REMINDERS

For The Morning...
Continuing your dry fast from your night sleep is a good idea. Work towards fasting up until at least 12pm. As your body adapts, start to increase this - the later you break your fast - the better.

In The Afternoon...
When you do finally decide to open your fast - focus on hydration. Spring water is a good start or slow-juiced fruits (e.g. berries, melons, citrus). Alternatively, eating soaked dates or your favourite fruits will suffice.

Evening Feast...
Work towards dry fasting for 23 hours and eating for 1 hour each day. This will take time to reach - listen to your body and get there in your own pace. The ideal time to break your dry fast would be approximately 6pm to 7pm

And At Night Time...
Be sure to completely stop eating by 8pm (latest) so your body can prepare for a good night's sleep, rest and recovery.

"Eat melons/ watermelons separately, and before any other fruit as they digest faster and we want to limit fermentation (acidity) which can occur if other fruits are mixed in."

DAY STRUCTURE REMINDERS

For The Morning...

Continuing your dry fast from your night sleep is a good idea. Work towards fasting up until at least 12pm. As your body adapts, start to increase this - the later you break your fast - the better.

In The Afternoon...

When you do finally decide to open your fast - focus on hydration. Spring water is a good start or slow-juiced fruits (e.g. berries, melons, citrus). Alternatively, eating soaked dates or your favourite fruits will suffice.

Evening Feast...

Work towards dry fasting for 23 hours and eating for 1 hour each day. This will take time to reach - listen to your body and get there in your own pace. The ideal time to break your dry fast would be approximately 6pm to 7pm

And At Night Time...

Be sure to completely stop eating by 8pm (latest) so your body can prepare for a good night's sleep, rest and recovery.

"Stay focussed on the end goal of removing mucus & toxins from your body and feeling wonderful! Look forward to being full of vitality and dis-ease free once again"

DAY STRUCTURE REMINDERS

For The Morning...

Continuing your dry fast from your night sleep is a good idea. Work towards fasting up until at least 12pm. As your body adapts, start to increase this - the later you break your fast - the better.

In The Afternoon...

When you do finally decide to open your fast - focus on hydration. Spring water is a good start or slow-juiced fruits (e.g. berries, melons, citrus). Alternatively, eating soaked dates or your favourite fruits will suffice.

Evening Feast...

Work towards dry fasting for 23 hours and eating for 1 hour each day. This will take time to reach - listen to your body and get there in your own pace. The ideal time to break your dry fast would be approximately 6pm to 7pm

And At Night Time...

Be sure to completely stop eating by 8pm (latest) so your body can prepare for a good night's sleep, rest and recovery.

"Meditate and perform deep breathing exercises in order to help yourself remain present minded and on track. Perform these techniques throughout the day but also during any challenging times that you may come to face."

DAY STRUCTURE REMINDERS

For The Morning...

Continuing your dry fast from your night sleep is a good idea. Work towards fasting up until at least 12pm. As your body adapts, start to increase this - the later you break your fast - the better.

In The Afternoon...

When you do finally decide to open your fast - focus on hydration. Spring water is a good start or slow-juiced fruits (e.g. berries, melons, citrus). Alternatively, eating soaked dates or your favourite fruits will suffice.

Evening Feast...

Work towards dry fasting for 23 hours and eating for 1 hour each day. This will take time to reach - listen to your body and get there in your own pace. The ideal time to break your dry fast would be approximately 6pm to 7pm

And At Night Time...

Be sure to completely stop eating by 8pm (latest) so your body can prepare for a good night's sleep, rest and recovery.

DAY 6: DAILY TIP

"Join a few like-minded communities – there are many juicing and raw vegan based groups, both online and offline. Being part of a community can help motivate you to reach your goals. You will also learn a great amount from others. Seeing others succeed is empowering."

DAY STRUCTURE REMINDERS

For The Morning...
Continuing your dry fast from your night sleep is a good idea. Work towards fasting up until at least 12pm. As your body adapts, start to increase this - the later you break your fast - the better.

In The Afternoon...
When you do finally decide to open your fast - focus on hydration. Spring water is a good start or slow-juiced fruits (e.g. berries, melons, citrus). Alternatively, eating soaked dates or your favourite fruits will suffice.

Evening Feast...
Work towards dry fasting for 23 hours and eating for 1 hour each day. This will take time to reach - listen to your body and get there in your own pace. The ideal time to break your dry fast would be approximately 6pm to 7pm

And At Night Time...
Be sure to completely stop eating by 8pm (latest) so your body can prepare for a good night's sleep, rest and recovery.

"If you are struggling to cope with hunger pangs in the early stages, try some dates or dried apricots, prunes, or raisins, with a cup of herbal tea. However, these pangs will disappear once your body adjusts to your new routine."

DAY STRUCTURE REMINDERS

For The Morning...
Continuing your dry fast from your night sleep is a good idea. Work towards fasting up until at least 12pm. As your body adapts, start to increase this - the later you break your fast - the better.

In The Afternoon...
When you do finally decide to open your fast - focus on hydration. Spring water is a good start or slow-juiced fruits (e.g. berries, melons, citrus). Alternatively, eating soaked dates or your favourite fruits will suffice.

Evening Feast...
Work towards dry fasting for 23 hours and eating for 1 hour each day. This will take time to reach - listen to your body and get there in your own pace. The ideal time to break your dry fast would be approximately 6pm to 7pm

And At Night Time...
Be sure to completely stop eating by 8pm (latest) so your body can prepare for a good night's sleep, rest and recovery.

"Get into a routine of regularly buying fresh fruit (or grow your own if weather permits) to keep your supplies up. Local wholesale markets do also clear fruit on Fridays (if they are closed for the weekend) at a lower price, so they are worth a visit."

DAY STRUCTURE REMINDERS

For The Morning...
Continuing your dry fast from your night sleep is a good idea. Work towards fasting up until at least 12pm. As your body adapts, start to increase this - the later you break your fast - the better.

In The Afternoon...
When you do finally decide to open your fast - focus on hydration. Spring water is a good start or slow-juiced fruits (e.g. berries, melons, citrus). Alternatively, eating soaked dates or your favourite fruits will suffice.

Evening Feast...
Work towards dry fasting for 23 hours and eating for 1 hour each day. This will take time to reach - listen to your body and get there in your own pace. The ideal time to break your dry fast would be approximately 6pm to 7pm

And At Night Time...
Be sure to completely stop eating by 8pm (latest) so your body can prepare for a good night's sleep, rest and recovery.

"Regularly remind yourself about the great rewards and benefits that you will experience by keeping up this detoxification process. Imagine the lives you could save as a result of healing yourself."

DAY STRUCTURE REMINDERS

For The Morning...

Continuing your dry fast from your night sleep is a good idea. Work towards fasting up until at least 12pm. As your body adapts, start to increase this - the later you break your fast - the better.

In The Afternoon...

When you do finally decide to open your fast - focus on hydration. Spring water is a good start or slow-juiced fruits (e.g. berries, melons, citrus). Alternatively, eating soaked dates or your favourite fruits will suffice.

Evening Feast...

Work towards dry fasting for 23 hours and eating for 1 hour each day. This will take time to reach - listen to your body and get there in your own pace. The ideal time to break your dry fast would be approximately 6pm to 7pm

And At Night Time...

Be sure to completely stop eating by 8pm (latest) so your body can prepare for a good night's sleep, rest and recovery.

"Keep your teeth brushed and flossed regularly – at least twice a day (morning & night) to keep them healthy for your fruit sessions. You will notice an improvement in your dental health with this raw/fruit diet."

DAY STRUCTURE REMINDERS

For The Morning...

Continuing your dry fast from your night sleep is a good idea. Work towards fasting up until at least 12pm. As your body adapts, start to increase this - the later you break your fast - the better.

In The Afternoon...

When you do finally decide to open your fast - focus on hydration. Spring water is a good start or slow-juiced fruits (e.g. berries, melons, citrus). Alternatively, eating soaked dates or your favourite fruits will suffice.

Evening Feast...

Work towards dry fasting for 23 hours and eating for 1 hour each day. This will take time to reach - listen to your body and get there in your own pace. The ideal time to break your dry fast would be approximately 6pm to 7pm

And At Night Time...

Be sure to completely stop eating by 8pm (latest) so your body can prepare for a good night's sleep, rest and recovery.

"Be motivated by the vision of becoming an example for others to learn from and follow. You could change the lives of family and friends by showing them your own improvements."

DAY STRUCTURE REMINDERS

For The Morning...

Continuing your dry fast from your night sleep is a good idea. Work towards fasting up until at least 12pm. As your body adapts, start to increase this - the later you break your fast - the better.

In The Afternoon...

When you do finally decide to open your fast - focus on hydration. Spring water is a good start or slow-juiced fruits (e.g. berries, melons, citrus). Alternatively, eating soaked dates or your favourite fruits will suffice.

Evening Feast...

Work towards dry fasting for 23 hours and eating for 1 hour each day. This will take time to reach - listen to your body and get there in your own pace. The ideal time to break your dry fast would be approximately 6pm to 7pm

And At Night Time...

Be sure to completely stop eating by 8pm (latest) so your body can prepare for a good night's sleep, rest and recovery.

"Embrace your achievements and wonderful results – feel and appreciate the difference within you as a result of this new routine. Notice how your personal agility and fitness has improved. Feel the improved energy levels."

DAY STRUCTURE REMINDERS

For The Morning...
Continuing your dry fast from your night sleep is a good idea. Work towards fasting up until at least 12pm. As your body adapts, start to increase this - the later you break your fast - the better.

In The Afternoon...
When you do finally decide to open your fast - focus on hydration. Spring water is a good start or slow-juiced fruits (e.g. berries, melons, citrus). Alternatively, eating soaked dates or your favourite fruits will suffice.

Evening Feast...
Work towards dry fasting for 23 hours and eating for 1 hour each day. This will take time to reach - listen to your body and get there in your own pace. The ideal time to break your dry fast would be approximately 6pm to 7pm

And At Night Time...
Be sure to completely stop eating by 8pm (latest) so your body can prepare for a good night's sleep, rest and recovery.

"Buy fruit in bulk where possible so you have ample supplies for a week or two in advance. If in a hot climate, you could even freeze your fruit or make ice lollies out of it (crush & freeze). Immerse yourself in fruit so it becomes your only option."

DAY STRUCTURE REMINDERS

For The Morning...
Continuing your dry fast from your night sleep is a good idea. Work towards fasting up until at least 12pm. As your body adapts, start to increase this - the later you break your fast - the better.

In The Afternoon...
When you do finally decide to open your fast - focus on hydration. Spring water is a good start or slow-juiced fruits (e.g. berries, melons, citrus). Alternatively, eating soaked dates or your favourite fruits will suffice.

Evening Feast...
Work towards dry fasting for 23 hours and eating for 1 hour each day. This will take time to reach - listen to your body and get there in your own pace. The ideal time to break your dry fast would be approximately 6pm to 7pm

And At Night Time...
Be sure to completely stop eating by 8pm (latest) so your body can prepare for a good night's sleep, rest and recovery.

"Stay as busy as you can during the daytime. Creating a busy routine makes it easier to manage your diet. Keep setting yourself new tasks/actions in order to keep yourself occupied."

DAY STRUCTURE REMINDERS

For The Morning...

Continuing your dry fast from your night sleep is a good idea. Work towards fasting up until at least 12pm. As your body adapts, start to increase this - the later you break your fast - the better.

In The Afternoon...

When you do finally decide to open your fast - focus on hydration. Spring water is a good start or slow-juiced fruits (e.g. berries, melons, citrus). Alternatively, eating soaked dates or your favourite fruits will suffice.

Evening Feast...

Work towards dry fasting for 23 hours and eating for 1 hour each day. This will take time to reach - listen to your body and get there in your own pace. The ideal time to break your dry fast would be approximately 6pm to 7pm

And At Night Time...

Be sure to completely stop eating by 8pm (latest) so your body can prepare for a good night's sleep, rest and recovery.

"Complete your fruit and fasting routine with a group of friends/family/colleagues so you can all support one another. Make it fun - set challenges - dry fast together and break your fasts together - have weekly catch up sessions."

DAY STRUCTURE REMINDERS

For The Morning...
Continuing your dry fast from your night sleep is a good idea. Work towards fasting up until at least 12pm. As your body adapts, start to increase this - the later you break your fast - the better.

In The Afternoon...
When you do finally decide to open your fast - focus on hydration. Spring water is a good start or slow-juiced fruits (e.g. berries, melons, citrus). Alternatively, eating soaked dates or your favourite fruits will suffice.

Evening Feast...
Work towards dry fasting for 23 hours and eating for 1 hour each day. This will take time to reach - listen to your body and get there in your own pace. The ideal time to break your dry fast would be approximately 6pm to 7pm

And At Night Time...
Be sure to completely stop eating by 8pm (latest) so your body can prepare for a good night's sleep, rest and recovery.

"Monitor your urine regularly in order to ensure your kidneys are filtering. Dry fasting for over 18 hours will increase kidney filtration. You can also drink the juice of slow-juiced citrus fruits (lemons, oranges). Sweating helps too."

DAY STRUCTURE REMINDERS

For The Morning...

Continuing your dry fast from your night sleep is a good idea. Work towards fasting up until at least 12pm. As your body adapts, start to increase this - the later you break your fast - the better.

In The Afternoon...

When you do finally decide to open your fast - focus on hydration. Spring water is a good start or slow-juiced fruits (e.g. berries, melons, citrus). Alternatively, eating soaked dates or your favourite fruits will suffice.

Evening Feast...

Work towards dry fasting for 23 hours and eating for 1 hour each day. This will take time to reach - listen to your body and get there in your own pace. The ideal time to break your dry fast would be approximately 6pm to 7pm

And At Night Time...

Be sure to completely stop eating by 8pm (latest) so your body can prepare for a good night's sleep, rest and recovery.

"Have genuine love and care for yourself. If you are craving junk food, affirm positive inner talk ("I won't feel good after eating junk. I love myself too much to put my body through that. So leave it out!"). You can also take Sea Kelp to reduce any salt cravings."

DAY STRUCTURE REMINDERS

For The Morning...
Continuing your dry fast from your night sleep is a good idea. Work towards fasting up until at least 12pm. As your body adapts, start to increase this - the later you break your fast - the better.

In The Afternoon...
When you do finally decide to open your fast - focus on hydration. Spring water is a good start or slow-juiced fruits (e.g. berries, melons, citrus). Alternatively, eating soaked dates or your favourite fruits will suffice.

Evening Feast...
Work towards dry fasting for 23 hours and eating for 1 hour each day. This will take time to reach - listen to your body and get there in your own pace. The ideal time to break your dry fast would be approximately 6pm to 7pm

And At Night Time...
Be sure to completely stop eating by 8pm (latest) so your body can prepare for a good night's sleep, rest and recovery.

"Feel and note down the difference within yourself as you filter out unwanted acids with this alkaline, water-dense fruits protocol."

DAY STRUCTURE REMINDERS

For The Morning...

Continuing your dry fast from your night sleep is a good idea. Work towards fasting up until at least 12pm. As your body adapts, start to increase this - the later you break your fast - the better.

In The Afternoon...

When you do finally decide to open your fast - focus on hydration. Spring water is a good start or slow-juiced fruits (e.g. berries, melons, citrus). Alternatively, eating soaked dates or your favourite fruits will suffice.

Evening Feast...

Work towards dry fasting for 23 hours and eating for 1 hour each day. This will take time to reach - listen to your body and get there in your own pace. The ideal time to break your dry fast would be approximately 6pm to 7pm

And At Night Time...

Be sure to completely stop eating by 8pm (latest) so your body can prepare for a good night's sleep, rest and recovery.

"Look out for white cloud/sediment (acids) in your urine to confirm that your kidneys are filtering out waste. Urinate in a glass jar - leave for 2 hours to settle before observing."

DAY STRUCTURE REMINDERS

For The Morning...
Continuing your dry fast from your night sleep is a good idea. Work towards fasting up until at least 12pm. As your body adapts, start to increase this - the later you break your fast - the better.

In The Afternoon...
When you do finally decide to open your fast - focus on hydration. Spring water is a good start or slow-juiced fruits (e.g. berries, melons, citrus). Alternatively, eating soaked dates or your favourite fruits will suffice.

Evening Feast...
Work towards dry fasting for 23 hours and eating for 1 hour each day. This will take time to reach - listen to your body and get there in your own pace. The ideal time to break your dry fast would be approximately 6pm to 7pm

And At Night Time...
Be sure to completely stop eating by 8pm (latest) so your body can prepare for a good night's sleep, rest and recovery.

"Infections emerge in an acidic environment. In order to remove infections, you must concentrate on kidney filtration. Use kidney (and adrenal) glandulars and dry fasting to assist."

DAY STRUCTURE REMINDERS

For The Morning...

Continuing your dry fast from your night sleep is a good idea. Work towards fasting up until at least 12pm. As your body adapts, start to increase this - the later you break your fast - the better.

In The Afternoon...

When you do finally decide to open your fast - focus on hydration. Spring water is a good start or slow-juiced fruits (e.g. berries, melons, citrus). Alternatively, eating soaked dates or your favourite fruits will suffice.

Evening Feast...

Work towards dry fasting for 23 hours and eating for 1 hour each day. This will take time to reach - listen to your body and get there in your own pace. The ideal time to break your dry fast would be approximately 6pm to 7pm

And At Night Time...

Be sure to completely stop eating by 8pm (latest) so your body can prepare for a good night's sleep, rest and recovery.

"Any deficiencies that you may have will start to disappear once you have cleansed your congested gut/colon, kidneys and various other eliminative organs."

DAY STRUCTURE REMINDERS

For The Morning...

Continuing your dry fast from your night sleep is a good idea. Work towards fasting up until at least 12pm. As your body adapts, start to increase this - the later you break your fast - the better.

In The Afternoon...

When you do finally decide to open your fast - focus on hydration. Spring water is a good start or slow-juiced fruits (e.g. berries, melons, citrus). Alternatively, eating soaked dates or your favourite fruits will suffice.

Evening Feast...

Work towards dry fasting for 23 hours and eating for 1 hour each day. This will take time to reach - listen to your body and get there in your own pace. The ideal time to break your dry fast would be approximately 6pm to 7pm

And At Night Time...

Be sure to completely stop eating by 8pm (latest) so your body can prepare for a good night's sleep, rest and recovery.

DAY 22: DAILY TIP

"Dependant on how deeply you detoxify yourself, it is possible to eliminate any genetic weaknesses that you may have inherited. This will require a deep detoxification process which involves juicing your fruits with prolonged periods of dry fasting"

DAY STRUCTURE REMINDERS

For The Morning...
Continuing your dry fast from your night sleep is a good idea. Work towards fasting up until at least 12pm. As your body adapts, start to increase this - the later you break your fast - the better.

In The Afternoon...
When you do finally decide to open your fast - focus on hydration. Spring water is a good start or slow-juiced fruits (e.g. berries, melons, citrus). Alternatively, eating soaked dates or your favourite fruits will suffice.

Evening Feast...
Work towards dry fasting for 23 hours and eating for 1 hour each day. This will take time to reach - listen to your body and get there in your own pace. The ideal time to break your dry fast would be approximately 6pm to 7pm

And At Night Time...
Be sure to completely stop eating by 8pm (latest) so your body can prepare for a good night's sleep, rest and recovery.

"Stay focused on your detoxification for deeper, lasting results. All past injuries / trauma are also repairable for good. Get those old acids out and replace them with a pain-free alkaline environment"

DAY STRUCTURE REMINDERS

For The Morning...

Continuing your dry fast from your night sleep is a good idea. Work towards fasting up until at least 12pm. As your body adapts, start to increase this - the later you break your fast - the better.

In The Afternoon...

When you do finally decide to open your fast - focus on hydration. Spring water is a good start or slow-juiced fruits (e.g. berries, melons, citrus). Alternatively, eating soaked dates or your favourite fruits will suffice.

Evening Feast...

Work towards dry fasting for 23 hours and eating for 1 hour each day. This will take time to reach - listen to your body and get there in your own pace. The ideal time to break your dry fast would be approximately 6pm to 7pm

And At Night Time...

Be sure to completely stop eating by 8pm (latest) so your body can prepare for a good night's sleep, rest and recovery.

"If you suffer from ongoing sadness / depression, a deep detox will support your mental health. You will soon notice a positive change in your mood.
Note: *you will need to support your adrenal glands and kidneys with glandulars and/or herbs"*

DAY STRUCTURE REMINDERS

For The Morning...
Continuing your dry fast from your night sleep is a good idea. Work towards fasting up until at least 12pm. As your body adapts, start to increase this - the later you break your fast - the better.

In The Afternoon...
When you do finally decide to open your fast - focus on hydration. Spring water is a good start or slow-juiced fruits (e.g. berries, melons, citrus). Alternatively, eating soaked dates or your favourite fruits will suffice.

Evening Feast...
Work towards dry fasting for 23 hours and eating for 1 hour each day. This will take time to reach - listen to your body and get there in your own pace. The ideal time to break your dry fast would be approximately 6pm to 7pm

And At Night Time...
Be sure to completely stop eating by 8pm (latest) so your body can prepare for a good night's sleep, rest and recovery.

"Have your fruits/ juices throughout the day - with dry fasting gaps of at least 3 hours in-between each feed. As the evening approaches, start to dry fast fully – from this point on, your body wants to rest and heal."

DAY STRUCTURE REMINDERS

For The Morning...
Continuing your dry fast from your night sleep is a good idea. Work towards fasting up until at least 12pm. As your body adapts, start to increase this - the later you break your fast - the better.

In The Afternoon...
When you do finally decide to open your fast - focus on hydration. Spring water is a good start or slow-juiced fruits (e.g. berries, melons, citrus). Alternatively, eating soaked dates or your favourite fruits will suffice.

Evening Feast...
Work towards dry fasting for 23 hours and eating for 1 hour each day. This will take time to reach - listen to your body and get there in your own pace. The ideal time to break your dry fast would be approximately 6pm to 7pm

And At Night Time...
Be sure to completely stop eating by 8pm (latest) so your body can prepare for a good night's sleep, rest and recovery.

"The kidneys dislike proteins but really appreciate juicy fruits like melons, berries, citrus fruits, pineapples, mangoes, apples, grapes. Witness the difference by replacing cooked foods and protein with fruits. Become the change."

DAY STRUCTURE REMINDERS

For The Morning...

Continuing your dry fast from your night sleep is a good idea. Work towards fasting up until at least 12pm. As your body adapts, start to increase this - the later you break your fast - the better.

In The Afternoon...

When you do finally decide to open your fast - focus on hydration. Spring water is a good start or slow-juiced fruits (e.g. berries, melons, citrus). Alternatively, eating soaked dates or your favourite fruits will suffice.

Evening Feast...

Work towards dry fasting for 23 hours and eating for 1 hour each day. This will take time to reach - listen to your body and get there in your own pace. The ideal time to break your dry fast would be approximately 6pm to 7pm

And At Night Time...

Be sure to completely stop eating by 8pm (latest) so your body can prepare for a good night's sleep, rest and recovery.

"Healing is very easy. There's no need to complicate it. Keep everything simple and you will see results. Concentrate on improving your level of health to a point where dis-ease is dissolved"

DAY STRUCTURE REMINDERS

For The Morning...
Continuing your dry fast from your night sleep is a good idea. Work towards fasting up until at least 12pm. As your body adapts, start to increase this - the later you break your fast - the better.

In The Afternoon...
When you do finally decide to open your fast - focus on hydration. Spring water is a good start or slow-juiced fruits (e.g. berries, melons, citrus). Alternatively, eating soaked dates or your favourite fruits will suffice.

Evening Feast...
Work towards dry fasting for 23 hours and eating for 1 hour each day. This will take time to reach - listen to your body and get there in your own pace. The ideal time to break your dry fast would be approximately 6pm to 7pm

And At Night Time...
Be sure to completely stop eating by 8pm (latest) so your body can prepare for a good night's sleep, rest and recovery.

"Keep your body in an alkaline and hydrated state as this is where regeneration takes place - and disease cannot continue to exist. You can achieve this through a raw fruits and vegetables diet (find your balance between the two)"

DAY STRUCTURE REMINDERS

For The Morning...
Continuing your dry fast from your night sleep is a good idea. Work towards fasting up until at least 12pm. As your body adapts, start to increase this - the later you break your fast - the better.

In The Afternoon...
When you do finally decide to open your fast - focus on hydration. Spring water is a good start or slow-juiced fruits (e.g. berries, melons, citrus). Alternatively, eating soaked dates or your favourite fruits will suffice.

Evening Feast...
Work towards dry fasting for 23 hours and eating for 1 hour each day. This will take time to reach - listen to your body and get there in your own pace. The ideal time to break your dry fast would be approximately 6pm to 7pm

And At Night Time...
Be sure to completely stop eating by 8pm (latest) so your body can prepare for a good night's sleep, rest and recovery.

"A daily enema with boiled water (cooled down) will support your detox greatly. Do not however become dependant on enemas, so after the initial week, start to wean yourself off."

DAY STRUCTURE REMINDERS

For The Morning...
Continuing your dry fast from your night sleep is a good idea. Work towards fasting up until at least 12pm. As your body adapts, start to increase this - the later you break your fast - the better.

In The Afternoon...
When you do finally decide to open your fast - focus on hydration. Spring water is a good start or slow-juiced fruits (e.g. berries, melons, citrus). Alternatively, eating soaked dates or your favourite fruits will suffice.

Evening Feast...
Work towards dry fasting for 23 hours and eating for 1 hour each day. This will take time to reach - listen to your body and get there in your own pace. The ideal time to break your dry fast would be approximately 6pm to 7pm

And At Night Time...
Be sure to completely stop eating by 8pm (latest) so your body can prepare for a good night's sleep, rest and recovery.

"Have your iris' read by an iridologist that works with Dr Bernard Jensen's system. An Iris Diagnosis will offer you information on specific areas of weakness that you can focus on"